Spa Bliss

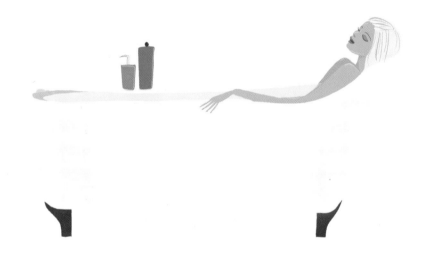

Spa Bliss

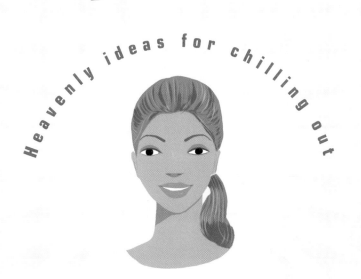

Heavenly ideas for chilling out

JO GLANVILLE-BLACKBURN

DUNCAN BAIRD PUBLISHERS

LONDON

Spa Bliss
Jo Glanville-Blackburn

Distributed in the USA and Canada by
Sterling Publishing Co., Inc.
387 Park Avenue South
New York, NY 10016-8810

This edition first published in the UK and USA in 2008 by
Duncan Baird Publishers Ltd
Sixth Floor, Castle House
75–76 Wells Street
London W1T 3QH

Managing Editor: Grace Cheetham
Editors: Dawn Bates, Zoë Fargher and Alison Bolus
Managing Designer: Daniel Sturges
Designer: Rebecca Johns
Commissioned colour artwork: Lucy Truman
Commissioned line artwork: Asami Mitsuhira for 3+Co.

For my family: my husband Jim Stanton and my darling children,
Olivia, William and Phoebe – without whom a 'home' spa – simply
becomes just a bathroom.

Library of Congress Cataloging-in-Publication Data Available

10 9 8 7 6 5 4 3 2 1

ISBN-13: 978-1-84483-522-5
ISBN-10: 1-84483-522-7

Typeset in Eurostile and Trade Gothic
Color reproduction by Colourscan, Singapore
Printed in China

For information about custom editions, special sales, premium
and corporate purchases, please contact Sterling Special Sales
Department at 800-805-5489 or specialsales@sterlingpub.com.

Publisher's note: The information in this book is not intended
as a substitute for professional medical advice and treatment.
If you are pregnant or are suffering from any medical conditions
or health problems, it is recommended that you consult a medical
professional before following any of the advice or practice
suggested in this book. Duncan Baird Publishers, or any other
persons who have been involved in working on this publication,
cannot accept responsibility for any injuries or damage incurred
as a result of following the information, recipes, exercises or
therapeutic techniques contained in this book.

Notes on the recipes
Unless otherwise stated:
• Do not mix metric and imperial measurements
• 1 tsp = 5ml, 1 tbsp = 15ml, 1 cup = 240ml

Contents

Introduction

Perhaps there is a good reason why the word "spa" rhymes with "aah". Spas are places we go to for total relaxation, where we can focus on ourselves and become gorgeous in the process, enjoying everything from the real basics, such as massages and manicures, to more exotic treatments, such as volcanic mud baths and seaweed body wraps. The beauty of this book is that you don't even have to leave your home to enjoy the spa experience.

Spa Bliss is the result of more than 20 years of my personal spa experiences, and includes all the most relaxing, restful spa rituals and routines I've found from Bali to Belfast. By including just a few of these in your lifestyle, you can turn a rushed health and beauty regime into a more holistic experience that will benefit your mind, body and soul. It is easy to recreate spa experiences at home. I once visited an Irish spa where the relaxation room had lovely, weighted lavender eye pillows. I bought a pair and since then have placed them over my eyes whenever I need a good night's sleep – the sensation immediately transports me straight back there.

I suggest you first read through the whole of Spa Bliss, turning down the corner of at least seven pages as you go; maybe you'll like the sound of the Hand massage, the Salt glow scrub or the Blissful spa bath. Pick out treatments you think you'll love, try some you think you might like and even one or two you think you might not like, just to see. The quick fixes will take you just five minutes, each daily routine lasts less than 15 minutes, and the weekend routines rarely take longer than half an hour.

Caring for yourself requires effort, time and a sense of self, and we often simply don't have the energy. Focusing completely on yourself and allowing yourself to be tremendously pampered helps you to shift your self-image and make a new start, so that you can begin to set aside some regular relaxation time. And once you have experienced the benefits of just a little extra attention, you'll be far less likely to ignore the needs of your mind and body in the future.

Prepare yourself

To benefit fully from your spa bliss experience, you need to set the scene. You can give yourself a face or body scrub any day of the year, but it's so much more rewarding with that spa touch. A good home spa treatment is as much about putting yourself in "the zone", using the exotic tropical aromas you'd find in a beautiful spa in Thailand or Bali to create an aura of calm and relaxation, as it is about what you put on your skin. So, turn up the heat, make a pile of fluffy towels, assemble essentials close to hand, and choose products or ingredients that evoke somewhere tropical and far, far away from home.

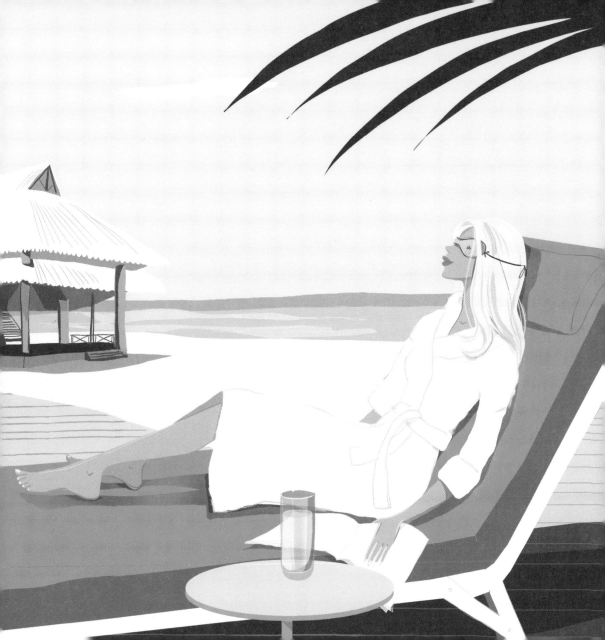

Secrets of the spa

Spas are based on the three Rs: rest, repair and replenishment of your mind, body and soul. The benefit of getting a good night's sleep is not a myth: your skin renews, repairs, cleanses and detoxifies itself between the hours of 10pm and 2am. With lack of sleep comes a lack of respite for your skin, and it will look progressively more exhausted, pale and dull. So many people skimp on sleep nowadays that beauty therapists are seeing an increased need for resurfacing, with body brushing and body scrubs, and hydration, using masks, wraps and thicker creams.

Help yourself to achieve a better state of health and vitality by recognizing your own innate need for rest and time to chill. Indulge in some relaxing and revitalizing spa rituals to help you to get 100 per cent back from your body, and you may find you can achieve everything more easily. So start now ...

◆ There are many ways to achieve as much rejuvenating rest as possible. One is to avoid stimulants such as coffee and alcohol after 6 o'clock in the evening. The toxins in these stimulants take time to break down, meaning that your body can't do its overnight job of cleansing and replenishing. Secondly, before going to bed, take a warm bath to relax your body and get you in the mood to sleep well. Finally, if you love and respect your body by giving it the attention it deserves, it will reward you in the long run. Pamper your skin, exercise your limbs and feed your mind, and you'll discover that it's easier to love yourself and to get a good night's sleep.

Recreate spa moments

Instead of spending a fortune at your local spa, why not try these simple steps for turning your own bathroom into a haven for balance, centring, healing, relaxation and renewal? It isn't difficult: all you have to do is treat your senses. Surround yourself with soothing colours, calming sounds and stimulating or relaxing textures, and you can make your bathroom into just the sanctuary you need for mind, body and soul.

◆ Few sounds are as calming as cascading water. Next time you fill a bath or run a shower, imagine it's a waterfall in a lush rainforest. When you turn off the water, welcome the quiet. Listening to music can soothe your senses, but just letting your mind be still can be wonderfully restorative too.

Cooling off with cold water on a hot day refreshes the senses, stimulates circulation and reduces inflammation. In contrast, warming up with a hot shower or bath on a cold day can be deeply nurturing and comforting. Some spa treatments take your body temperature from hot to cold and back to hot again, in order to stimulate the circulation and revitalize your skin.

Colour is very important and can be used to create or enhance a mood. Tranquil aquamarine and sky blue are great colours for a bathroom. In addition, green is a very healing colour, yellow soothes the nerves and violet encourages creativity, while pure, pristine white represents cleanliness. So, depending on the mood you want to evoke, go ahead and tint your bath water, use coloured towels or wrap up in your favourite-coloured bathrobe.

The path to bliss

While some forms of stress can be positive and creative, most are damaging, weakening our immune systems, robbing our bodies of vital life-giving nutrients and increasing the likelihood of illness while hindering recovery. If you are to avoid stress getting worse, it's vital to learn to recognize the early signs in your own body, such as headaches, neck and back pain, digestive disorders, fatigue or recurring colds and infections. Once you spot the telltale signals, enjoy a blissful de-stressing technique and, hopefully, your stress-related condition will pass or be prevented.

A balanced and positive attitude will also help to offset stress. Research shows that laughter is good for us, so smile as you get ready for some pampering. You can do several things in combination, or just pick and choose. That's what is great about a home spa: you can do whatever you want to feel good about yourself!

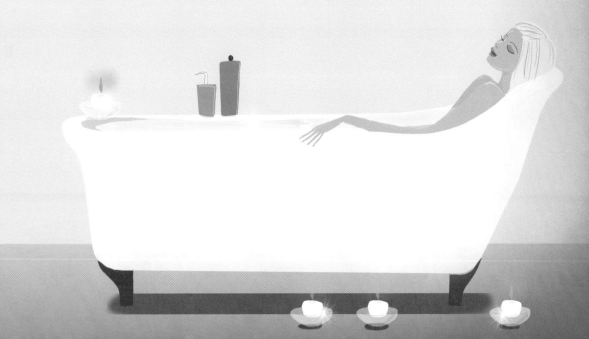

Create the perfect spa environment in your bathroom by lighting some candles and infusing the air using an essential oil burner (see page 17). Feng shui experts say that a lighted beeswax candle can increase the positive energy, or chi, in a room. Pot plants, meanwhile, will absorb carbon dioxide and replenish the oxygen in the air, so put one in the corner of the room. Collect shells, pebbles or stones, and display them: just looking at sea shells can open your mind for visualization (see page 102).

Stones and crystals are believed to hold vibrational energy and water has its own vibration, so the combination of the two is powerful. Simply add a crystal to your bathwater to try out the effects.

Aromatherapy to chill

Our sense of smell is very powerful. The principle of aromatherapy is that the fragrances of certain essential oils can have positive effects on our brains, the very nerve centres of our entire bodies and home to our every thought, feeling and emotion. Although we can't expect aromatherapy to fix the root of any emotional problems we might have, there's no doubt that the aroma of carefully chosen oils can help to support us in tough times or give us a comforting place to curl up in when we need security. So use aromatherapy to help you relax, de-stress, bliss out and create a feeling of total well-being.

An essential oil burner is vital for aromatherapy. Inexpensive burners are widely available, but why not buy a more attractive one that you can use as an item of decoration? You will be more likely to use it regularly.

Simply fill the well at the top of the burner with water, add a few drops of essential oil, light a candle underneath and let the heat warm the oil, filling the air with scent. You can also add a few drops of essential oil to unfragranced toiletries such as body lotion.

Essential oils

Essential oils to put you in a constant state of bliss include: bergamot, which has a pleasant, sweet and fruity smell, with stimulating anti-depressant properties; rose, which gives a sense of security and happiness (most women absolutely adore the sensual, feminine aroma of rose, which, mixed with geranium and a base oil, smells beautiful on the skin); rosewood, which is a lovely, sweet, woody fragrance that helps to treat stress, nervousness, anxiety and sadness; frankincense, which dispels bad moods and lifts the spirits; and sandalwood, which is a beautiful, soulful scent that calms and quietens a lively mind and enables us to find some inner peace. Orange, mandarin, lemon and lime are all popular essential oils (and inexpensive as they're easy to extract) that brighten a mood, ease tension and relieve sadness.

Add one drop of peppermint (to revive), lavender (to balance), rosemary (to clear the head) or geranium (to calm) essential oil to a tissue and hold it under your nose. Breathe deeply for a count of five, then remove the tissue. Repeat five times or as necessary.

To ease swelling or aches and pains, or to decongest areas of the body, apply a compress. Add five drops of essential oil to 250ml/9fl oz/1 cup of hot or cold water. Soak a facecloth in the liquid, squeeze out and apply to your skin.

Place some essential oils in a burner or in a bowl of hot water to fill the air with the wonderful aroma of your favourite choice of oils, and use it to influence your mood, create a relaxing ambience, revive flagging spirits and disperse unpleasant smells such as cigarette smoke.

Exotic spa ingredients

Every spa devotee knows that some of the best natural therapeutic ingredients are found growing in exotic locations. If you truly want to feel as if you've "got away from it all", you just need a handful of beautiful flowers and some deliciously fragrant oils, and you can recreate the smell and the atmosphere of a tropical island beach. Just lie back, close your eyes, inhale their gorgeous scent, and imagine yourself in paradise, bathed in warm sunshine and listening to the soft lapping of waves.

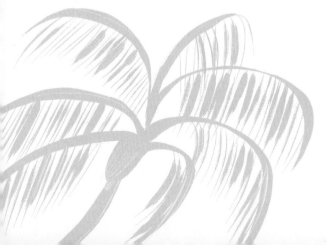

Coconut oil has one of the most recognizable and evocative of all tropical scents, and has been used for centuries in the Caribbean to soften skin. You can use coconut oil to moisturize dry lips, or massage it into other dry areas of the body. It is also effective as a hair mask. You can use coconut oil alone, or mix it with other oils or vegetable butters.

Cocoa butter, extracted from the cacao bean, is an inexpensive butter cream rich in nutrients and emollients, making it ideal for very dry skin on elbows, lower legs, heels and lips. Cacao beans, of course, also give us cocoa and chocolate, explaining cocoa butter's delicious, almost edible, fragrance.

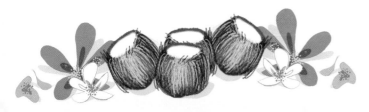

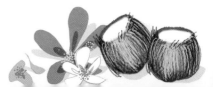

Explore your senses

Two of the most popular Hawaiian plant oils come from the macadamia nut and the kukui nut. More rare are the essential oils of Polynesia: Tahitian Tiare Gardenia, Pikake (jasmine), which yields a light but exquisite scent, and Plumeria (frangipani), which has a sweet, somewhat intoxicating scent. Easier to find, and easy to use whenever you're in the mood for a spa experience, versatile natural oils such as olive and almond, as well as richly aromatic spices such as ginger and cloves, feature in many spa bliss treatments, so stock up on them.

◆ You can use olive oil on your face, your body and even your hair. For a conditioning treatment, simply massage olive oil into your hair, wrap it in a warm towel and leave on for 20–60 minutes while you have a blissful bath. Shampoo well before rinsing out.

Almond oil is a great humectant (it keeps moisture in your skin), and makes a lovely body oil. You can use it alone or mix it with a few drops of your favourite essential oils to create aromatherapy blends. Of course, avoid almond oil if you are allergic to nuts.

Warming and stimulating, ginger raises the body temperature. Its hot, tingling flavour is often used to enhance the taste of herbal teas, drinks and, of course, Asian curries. However, it is also a lovely ingredient in body creams and has long been used as an aphrodisiac cream for brides in south Asia. Cloves also raise the body temperature and have a very distinctive, rich aroma.

Quick fix spa tricks

When you're short of time, try out these five-minute spa treats and rituals. Although they are quick, they really do make a difference. Even if you squeeze just one of these into your evening, every evening for a week, you will have pampered yourself for an extra half an hour that you wouldn't have done before.

You will soon find that just a little extra attention really does boost the way you look and the way you feel about yourself, both inside and out.

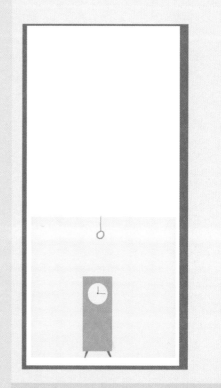

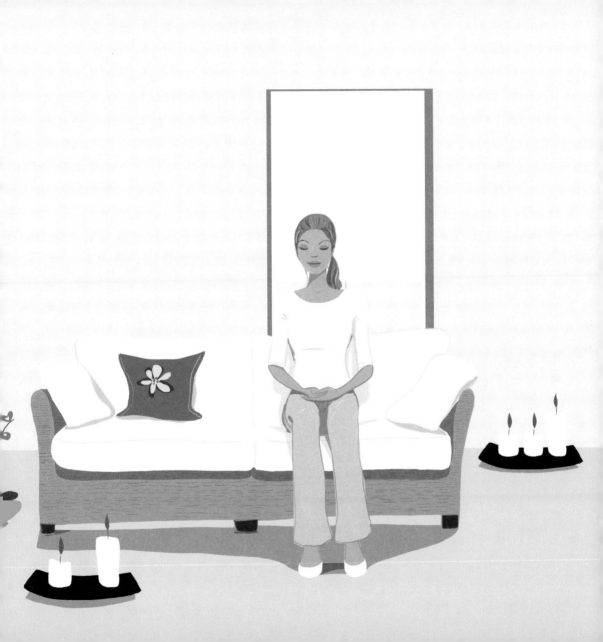

To relax

I always need to lie down to relax. We are all living lives under increasing pressure, and it's easy to perceive sleep as being less important than it is. The good news is that if you do need to skimp on your night-time sleep, experts say that a siesta-like "power nap" of five minutes during the day can reboot your mental alertness. Just think how those holiday afternoon snoozes restore body and soul. Likewise at a spa, it's the norm to cozy up after a massage and just chill out. So put yourself in this snooze mode. And even if you're not low on sleep, book in for the occasional restorative afternoon nap whenever you feel the need.

Make up a soporific aromatherapy blend of two drops of frankincense and one drop each of lavender, rose and sandalwood essential oils. Mix in two teaspoons of almond base oil and place a few drops on a clean handkerchief or paper tissue. Hold under your nose and take five slow, deep breaths. Also try spraying a relaxing aromatherapy scent on your pillowcases.

Lie down on your back, arms by your side, palms facing up. Focus on your breathing and be aware of the weight of your body becoming heavier and heavier, until you feel unable to move. Concentrate on your breathing for five minutes, then wriggle your toes and fingers, open your eyes and slowly come up to sitting.

To de-stress

Tension can be running through your body at any time of day. Without realizing it, you may be gritting your teeth, hunching your shoulders or frowning in concentration. Yet if you just relax your muscles, you can de-stress quickly and easily.

There are simple ways to de-stress while you are at home. To release tension in your neck, sit comfortably and lift your shoulders up to your ears. Hold for a few seconds, then lower again. Repeat three times. Then rock your head gently from side to side. Try breathing deeply: sit cross-legged with your back supported, close your eyes and place one hand on your abdomen and the other on your chest. Breathe in slowly and concentrate on moving only your lower hand. Do this for five minutes. To create a calm atmosphere, add two to three drops of balancing geranium essential oil to a bowl with a little warm water, and leave it to diffuse into the air.

◆ Wipe away tension from your brows with a quick but highly effective massage. Place a calming mix of two drops each of lavender and rose essential oil in two teaspoons of almond oil between your fingertips. Inhale a little of the oil, then place your middle fingers on the inner edge of each brow. Gently but firmly, brush along the length of your brows. Now, starting from the inner corners again, press several times to the ends. Brush again. Inhale once more and relax.

To restore

Soothe and restore yourself and feel renewed by carrying out some simple techniques at home that take just a few minutes. To stretch your spine – great for first thing in the morning – kneel on the floor and stretch your arms out in front of you until your forehead rests on the floor. Breathe slowly.

To restore great skin, fill a basin with hot water and dip a clean flannel or muslin facecloth in it. Wring through and, while still hot, wipe over areas of your skin. This draws out impurities and helps to minimize fine lines and wrinkles.

If you like a morning bath, a couple of handfuls of coarse sea salt thrown in the water will lightly scrub your skin and leave you feeling wonderfully revived. Alternatively, give yourself an invigorating skin rub while in the shower, or try changing the temperature of the water.

◆ Not enough sleep and a hard day at the office can leave you with puffy, tired and sore eyes. Restore them by soaking and chilling two tea bags, and placing the tea bags on closed eyelids for five minutes. The tannin in the tea will help to repair damaged skin cells, diminish dark circles and reduce puffiness.

Juicing

Fresh fruit and vegetable juices are an extremely effective way of absorbing large amounts of health-giving, anti-ageing nutrients and can be highly cleansing and detoxifying. Devotees of juicing believe that raw juice is the most perfect fuel for your body. Pure juices cleanse and nurture, while boosting your health with vitamins and minerals. However, if you remove the fibre (pulp) you will still need to eat fresh fruit and vegetables to obtain the required amount of roughage in your diet.

Some juices are associated with treating certain conditions: cranberry juice for cystitis; celery juice for fluid retention; leafy green vegetable juice for neutralizing toxins in the gut; and papaya and carrot juice for digestive problems.

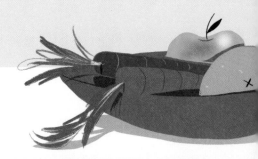

✦ For a delicious, cleansing drink that will soothe your
stomach and aid digestion, juice three apples, three
carrots and three pineapple rings together.

For an antioxidant skin booster, juice half a red pepper, half
a green pepper and half a cucumber separately from each other,
then mix. This juice is high in vitamins C, E and beta-carotene,
as well as zinc and potassium, which stimulate your digestive
system and kidneys to work efficiently.

Whenever you feel slightly tense or
need to unwind, juice a green apple with
two celery sticks and 10 lettuce leaves,
and drink before bedtime.

Daily routines

We all long to escape from the stresses of everyday life from time to time and, with a little know-how, you can do this easily at home. Even the most everyday spa-like rituals, such as a facial treatment or a body wrap, can make you feel blissfully pampered and nurtured.

Exotic aromas and ingredients can help to conjure up memories of spa days. Here I divulge spa secrets just for you, so that you can easily recreate them at home – and not one of these treatments will take longer than 15 minutes.

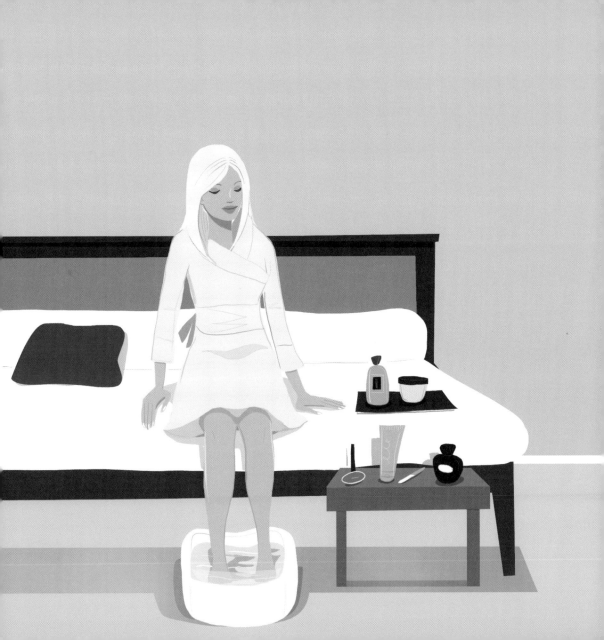

Everyday exfoliation

Few beauty treatments deliver such instantaneous results as a face scrub. Exfoliation is vital for brighter, fresher, vibrant-looking skin, as it boosts circulation and your skin's natural renewal processes, and removes dull-looking dead cells from your skin's surface to expose younger, fresher skin beneath. Done weekly, it also helps skin creams to penetrate faster and more effectively. Exfoliation is most effective, and rewarding, in the evening when your skin has had a chance to adapt to the atmosphere. In the morning, your skin may be less supple.

You can exfoliate using a grainy scrub, a buffing cloth (muslin or flannel) or a peel made from a fruit that contains naturally occurring protein-digestive enzymes, such as papaya (papain) or pineapple (bromelain). These gently but effectively dissolve dead skin cells, leaving skin brighter and smoother. Concentrate on your nose, chin and forehead, and avoid the area around your eyes. Moisturize afterwards.

✦ Mix one tablespoon each of coconut milk (to moisturize and soften your skin), mashed pineapple (to tackle dead skin cells) and plain yogurt (to balance your skin's acidity) with two tablespoons of honey, which has anti-bacterial and anti-inflammatory properties. Apply this mask to clean skin and leave on for 10 minutes. Rinse the mask off with cool water. You may not need to apply a moisturizer after this mask, because coconut milk is very hydrating and contains plenty of oil.

Steamy stuff

Steaming your face will help to open your pores and release any impurities, and the treatment is as simple as pouring hot water into a bowl. You may like to add some calming herbs such as chamomile, lavender or calendula (marigold) to the water. You could also add a couple of drops of rose or lavender essential oil (just two drops, as you don't want to irritate your eyes). If you have roses at home, you could also put rose petals into the water for a lovely scent.

Once you have steamed your face, your skin will have softened, so it is a great opportunity to clear blocked pores and extract any blackheads you may have. Afterwards, make a solution of three drops of lavender oil in a cup of water and dab onto your skin using a cottonwool pad.

⬥ First, thoroughly cleanse your skin, making sure that it is free of make-up. Work gently around your eyes, using a circular motion. Apply a face exfoliator and massage in with gentle circular movements, then rinse off with fresh water.

Pour about 1.25 litres/2 pints/ 5 cups of boiling water into a bowl. Put a towel over your head and lean forward with your face about 30cm/1ft over the bowl. You should feel comfortable,

although at times the steam may feel overpowering up your nose. If you feel a burning sensation, stop and wait for the water to cool a little. Once comfortable, steam for 10 minutes.

Body brushing blitz

This simple action of gentle skin brushing using a dry natural bristle brush can have magical effects on your skin. It stimulates circulation and buffs dead skin cells off the surface of your skin to leave it soft, gleaming and glowing, and prevent it drying out. Loved by the Russians and Scandinavians for centuries as part of their daily ablutions, dry body brushing also helps to stimulate the lymphatic system and so eliminates toxins through your skin, and is believed to help prevent and reduce the appearance of cellulite. Body brushing is a treatment that is offered in many spas.

Always brush your body with long, gentle strokes, starting at your feet and working upward toward your heart, as in a massage. From your hips and abdomen, move on to your fingers and gradually brush your way to your shoulders and across your chest, back and neck. Avoid your face and any areas that have cuts, broken capillaries or varicose veins.

Alternatively, a loofah is one of the cheapest and most convenient ways to scrub and can be used during the shower as a sponge. Let it dry after every use to avoid mould forming. Textured mitts or gloves made of natural materials such as sisal can also be used.

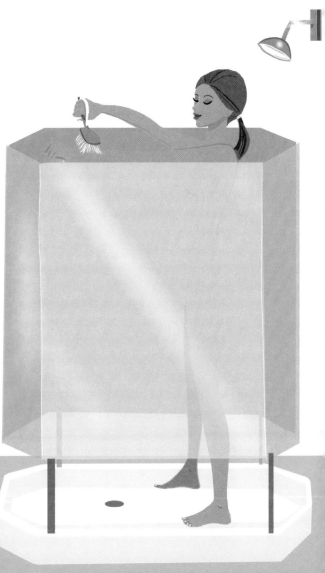

Salt glow scrub

Scrubs are as beneficial to your body as they are to your face, and spas around the world offer a large variety of exfoliating treatments. In most cultures, women have long used exfoliation as part of their daily bath or shower. Body scrubs clear the skin of dead cells and help its natural renewal processes. They help to remove bumpy skin (such as on the backs of your arms) and quickly give your whole body a refreshed appearance. Next time you shower, try the Caribbean salt glow scrub opposite, which will leave your skin smooth, soft and deliciously scented.

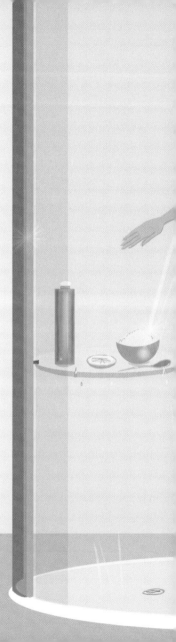

★ Mix 250ml/9fl oz/1 cup of a vegetable oil, such as almond or apricot, with one teaspoon of fresh lime juice and 15 drops in total of your chosen combination of lemon, grapefruit, ginger, neroli and ylang-ylang essential oils.

For a truly tropical spa sensation, add three tablespoons of coconut oil for extra moisture, which will also add a gorgeous beachy aroma to your treatment. Now mix in 250ml/9fl oz/1 cup of sea salt.

Stand in your shower or bath, wash yourself, then apply the mixture using your hands. Concentrate on exfoliating your upper back, shoulders, upper arms, bottom, elbows and knees, massaging in the scrub with gentle circular movements. Treat anywhere else on your body, including your hands and feet, with a lighter action. Rinse off.

Frown anti-age massage

Forget Botox: with a bit of practice, this blissfully soothing facial pressure-point massage will relieve tension and aid lymphatic drainage, giving your face an uplifted, youthful look. Either carry it out using a creamy cleanser or, if you prefer, do the massage in the evening using almond oil, or a blend of half a teaspoon of wheatgerm oil with one drop of rose oil if your skin feels dry.

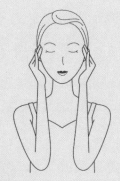

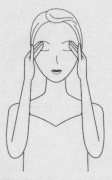

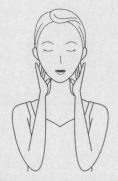

1 Use your fingers to smooth away any lines on your forehead with a gentle "press and release" action. Start at the bridge of your nose, press and release. Then glide up to the edge of your inner eyebrow, press and release, then to the outer edge of your brow. Move to your temples, feel for the fingertip-size dent, then press and release.

2 To lift your eyes, place your fingers under each eyebrow, then press and release. Glide up to your brows, press and release. Then do two more movements up your forehead toward your hairline.

3 To increase circulation and brighten your skin, massage outward from the centre of your face using light, sweeping movements. Move along your brow line to your temples, across your forehead to your temples, then from under your eyes, from the sides of your nose and finally from your chin to your ears.

* To finish your massage, lie back, close your eyes and place a soaked and chilled chamomile tea bag over each eyelid. Massage your temples for one minute.

Hair and scalp massage

During illness and times of stress or poor nutrition, your body conserves vital nutrients in order to cope. The first place it stops supplying is your skin, which, of course, includes your scalp. Not surprisingly, skin problems that are hidden under your hair can go unnoticed or be ignored for quite some time. But, ultimately, a healthy scalp means healthier, thicker, more lustrous hair, so it's a good idea to offer your scalp some love and attention from time to time.

Scalp massage is very stimulating and therapeutic, and will increase the blood flow to nerve endings and boost your scalp health. Relax and enjoy this soothing massage whenever you get the chance.

◆ Gently rub tiny circles along your shoulders and up the sides of your neck. Then press in tiny circles all along on either side of your hairline until you reach your centre parting. Now place all your fingers in your hair and gently massage your scalp in tiny circles and larger strokes. Finally, lift your hair upward in your hands, and pull very gently for a count of three. Repeat several times.

Try massaging your scalp using a stimulating blend of two teaspoons of castor oil or grapeseed oil and five drops of eucalyptus or rosemary oil. Massage it over your scalp, and leave on as long as possible. Rinse thoroughly.

Restful tummy massage

Abdominal massage eases tension and stimulates circulation, which can help with trapped wind, indigestion and the movement of waste to your colon. This technique is inspired by the Maya, who regularly performed tummy massages to improve digestion, correct digestion-related problems and relax the internal organs. A regular, gentle abdominal massage may help to soothe the digestive and reproductive organs in your lower abdomen. It's an ideal treatment if you often feel bloated or have gas, suffer from tummy aches or period pain, or find your appetite is poor. I like to precede a tummy massage with a hot water bottle, to warm my skin and ease any discomfort.

◆ Begin with a relaxing chest massage. Sitting upright, apply a massage oil such as almond oil across your chest in sweeping motions. One side at a time, work from your shoulders down to your pectoral (chest) muscles, gently squeezing between your fingers and the heel of your hand.

Then lie down and smooth oil over your abdomen. Massage in circular movements in a clockwise direction (following the direction of movement in your colon and to stimulate digestion). If you prefer, you can use smaller, wider or firmer strokes across your tummy: choose whatever feels most comforting.

Hand massage

Hands get stressed out too. In fact, I think a relaxing hand massage is the best part of any decent manicure. Use this as a time to deeply moisturize your hands, and to flex tense joints, especially if you use a computer frequently.

   You can use hand cream to massage your hands, but oil is better as it allows your hands to glide more easily over your skin. Choose from sweet almond, jojoba, avocado or apricot oil, and for extra therapeutic benefits, blend one of these base oils (or two or three of them) with your favourite essential oil. However, do bear in mind that your hands will be slippery afterwards, so I'd always recommend that you do a hand massage with oil last thing before bed.

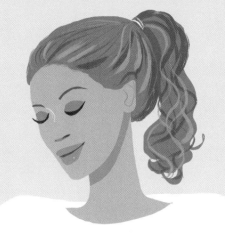

✦ Form your hands into two clenched fists, hold for a few seconds then straighten them out as you release. Repeat 10 times. Now clasp them together. Press your fingers together as hard as you can for a count of five. Shake your fingers out and repeat 10 times.

Place your palms together as if in prayer. Then lift your palms so that only your fingers and thumbs remain in contact with each other. Press for a count of three and release. Repeat 10 times.

Smooth oil all over your forearms and squeeze each arm. Then massage your hands, kneading each palm with the knuckles of your opposite hand. Finish by gently pulling each finger between your opposite thumb and forefinger, working from the joint to the fingertip.

Spa manicure

No spa session would be complete without a final buff and polish to the nails. It's as if we realize that while we may pummel, scrub and purge our bodies in an attempt to achieve a whole new self, a spa manicure can make at least our hands look gorgeous quickly and easily. It takes a bit of know-how, but a mini manicure can improve even the most dry and worn out of hands, so there's no excuse not to groom and pamper them.

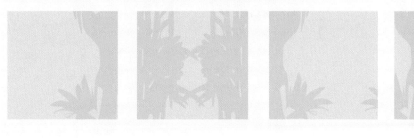

File your nails into shape with a soft emery board (avoid using a metal file, which may split your nails). Next, massage cuticle cream into the nail area, and place your fingertips in a bowl of warm, soapy water for two minutes to soften your cuticles.

Dry your hands and gently push back the cuticles with an orange stick. Now massage in a little cuticle oil (or almond oil) around the nail bed, followed by hand cream all over your hands and fingers.

Lightly buff the surface of your nails with a nail buffer, and rub them smooth using the softer side. Now your nails should look sleek, shiny and healthy, and are ready to be either left beautifully bare, or painted with polish.

Foot massage

We so rarely devote enough quality time to our feet, yet they can make such a difference to the way we feel. Just stroking your feet has a hugely uplifting effect on your whole body. One blissfully relaxing treat is to soak tired feet in a bowl of warm water with a couple of drops each of geranium and lavender essential oils. And whenever you get the chance, walk barefoot around your home for at least 10 minutes to allow your feet to spread. Try a refreshing blend of two drops of tea tree oil mixed with two teaspoons of almond oil for the massage opposite.

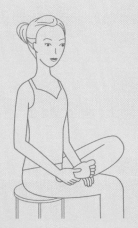 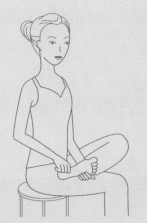 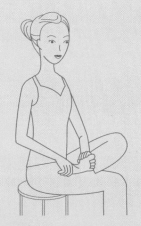

1 Warm a couple of drops of oil between the palms of your hands and smooth it over your left foot. Make long, firm thumb sweeps along the length of your sole from the arch to the toes.

2 Grasp your left foot with your left hand and rub the soles with the knuckles of your right hand. Make small circles with your thumbs, working from the ball of the foot to the heel.

3 Finally, hold the toes with one hand and the heel with the other and wring your foot by twisting your hands in opposite directions. Repeat all three exercises on your right foot

 If your feet are really dry, the best treatment is to smother them in foot cream or petroleum jelly and wear old socks overnight. While not recommended on hot summer nights, it's guaranteed to improve the driest of feet by morning.

Weekend routines

We're all busy being busy, but our bodies are crying out to be nurtured and cared for properly. These beauty techniques take a bit longer, so save them for your weekends, when you have a little more time to pamper without having to rush. To truly indulge yourself, switch off your phone, and turn off the TV and radio. If you want some sound, play soothing music. These peaceful, restful rituals will quickly help you to relax, unwind, and de-stress whenever you like — it's just up to you to make the time.

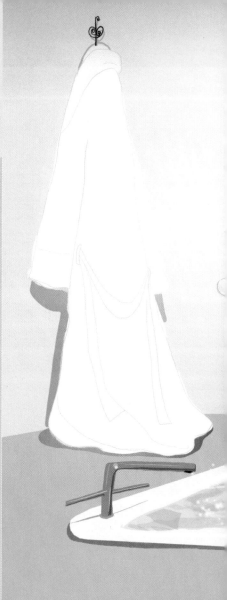

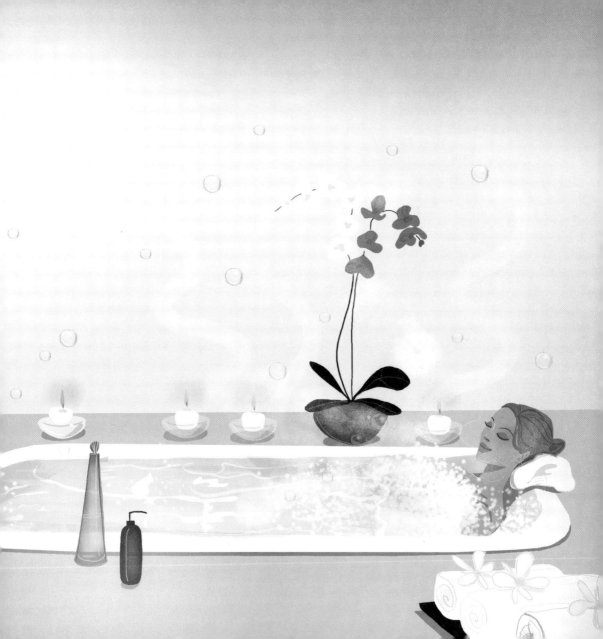

Facemasks

If there's one beauty treatment worth squeezing into your spa experience, it's a facemask. To benefit from a facemask, you need to leave it on your skin for a while, meaning you really have to stop, lie still and chill. So it's the perfect de-stress treatment, but best of all, a facemask will leave you feeling positively pampered.

If you're buying a ready-made mask, there's one to suit every need (see page 61), but if you're making your own, choose ingredients to suit your skin type. After all, few skins are oily or dry all over. Some people with oily skin get patchy zones of dehydration, while others have dry skin with an oily T-zone. The hydrating pumpkin mask opposite is perfect for dry skin. Pumpkin is rich in nutrients which will help to moisturize your skin and leave it soft and supple.

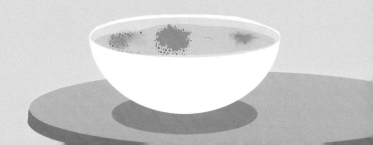

You will need three tablespoons of canned or cooked pumpkin, ¼ teaspoon of jojoba oil, ½ teaspoon of honey and ¼ teaspoon of milk (if you have normal or oily skin) or butter-milk (if you have dry skin). If you do have dry skin and do not suffer from breakouts, you can add a few drops of evening primrose oil from a cap-sule. Mix the ingredients together and apply to your face. Leave the facemask on for 15 minutes while you relax, then clean it off with lukewarm water.

Applying a facemask

If you are buying a facemask, select one that matches your needs. Many masks contain exotic flower or plant oils and/or herbal extracts to improve the skin's appearance. See the opposite page for the basic mask formulas you can buy.

Always cleanse your skin before applying a facemask – using a facemask on a dirty face is like putting polish on a dirty floor. Apply the mask to your face, lie down if you like and play some relaxing music. You could also place some soaked and chilled tea bags over your eyes. Leave the mask on for around 15 minutes (or however long instructed). Depending on the type of mask you chose, wash, peel or remove with a tissue. Then apply some toner and follow with your normal moisturizer.

◆ Clay-based masks for oily skin are smooth and thick in texture, and contain ingredients such as tar and seaweed extracts. They are often scented with stimulating menthol or camphor.

Peel-off masks help to remove dirt and impurities. They are usually light, and often dry in minutes. Moisturizing masks are rich and creamy, and soften signs of dehydration, ageing and tiredness.

Revitalizing masks refresh and brighten dull skin. They often contain vitamin C or exfoliants, and are perfect after a long day or before a party.

Moisture moment

Never skimp on moisturizing. Moisturizers for the face and body include antioxidant, protective, preventative and anti-ageing creams, but their basic function remains the same: to act as a barrier and keep moisture in the skin. Regularly assess your skin. If you are prone to blocked pores or blackheads, you probably have oily skin, and should switch to an oil-free moisturizer. In contrast, if your skin is dry, you need to up your water intake and choose a moisturizer that contains humectants (such as hyaluronic acid), which attract more water to your skin.

For plump, glowing, healthy-looking skin, apply moisturizer after every bath and shower, until it becomes routine. Moisturize from the inside, too, by getting into the habit of drinking water. Try drinking a glass of hot water with a slice of lemon instead of coffee or tea – it's refreshing, thirst-quenching and skin-replenishing.

This banana beauty balm is both cleansing and moisturizing. Mash two bananas in a bowl using a fork. Warm four tablespoons of whipping cream and four teaspoons of honey and add to the banana. Stir well. Add four drops of chamomile oil and one tablespoon of finely powdered oats and stir again. Apply this deep-moisturizing mask to clean skin and leave on for 10 minutes. Wipe the mask off with a clean tissue, then rinse with fresh water. Pat your skin dry, and follow with your daily moisturizer to keep your skin soft.

Blissful spa bath

Simply bathing is a much underrated mind and body therapy. Where else in the home can you be sure to find at least 20 minutes of peace and solitude, immersed in aromatic delights? There are so many different types of baths in the spa industry that collectively they're called "hydrotherapy" treatments. Try taking a blissful bath last thing at night, to "waft" in rather than to wash in. Think of it as a haven of pure relaxation, a treat for your body rather than simply a way to keep clean. Set the scene and dim the lights, then lie back, close your eyes and immerse yourself in delicious bath spa treats, using your favourite essential oils.

You can even meditate while you're in the tub. Roll up a towel under your neck, lie back and visualize waves lapping gently around your shoulders. Close your eyes and breathe slowly and deeply. Imagine that you are in a pool by the sea. Concentrate on your breathing and on the rhythm of the water rising and falling with each breath.

An aromatherapy bath is a great way to shift your mood. Many essential oils have therapeutic uses, so use them to relax your mind and muscles after a long day or a tiring workout. Add 6–10 drops of pure essential oil, or one or two capfuls of a pre-mixed blend (two or three drops of essential oils mixed together in a base oil), to the bath once the water has run, then lie back and enjoy.

Try this Spa Bliss Bath Blend: add two drops each of geranium, rose and mandarin essential oils in two table-spoons of almond oil. Soak for a full 20 minutes to totally bliss out.

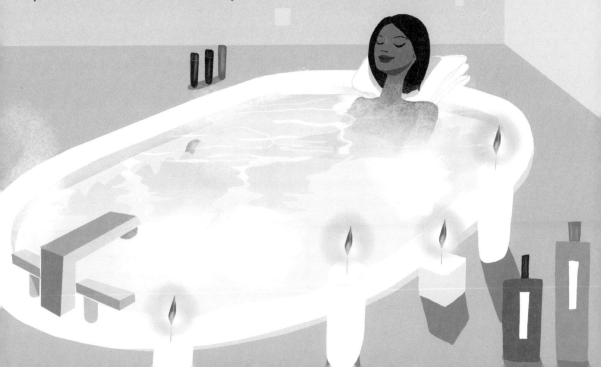

Tea-time bath

You can use everyday storecupboard ingredients to create a therapeutic spa-like bath. Drinking green tea has proven antioxidant anti-ageing effects, so why not also enjoy its health benefits by bathing in it, nourishing your skin from the outside? Relaxing, exotic and indulgent, a green tea bath leaves your skin beautifully soft.

Place two tablespoons each of loose green tea, peppermint tea, chamomile tea and oat flour in a bowl, then add five drops each of lavender and neroli essential oils. Mix the ingredients together, adding enough aloe vera juice or water to create a paste. Spread out a 15cm/6in diameter piece of muslin and add the paste to the centre of the cloth, then draw all the edges up together and tie the neck with a rubber band or piece of string. Hang the bag underneath your bath tap so that the water flows through it, then lie down and soak for 20 blissful minutes.

If you have dry, irritated skin, place two generous handfuls of oatmeal in your muslin bag, and squeeze it from time to time as the water runs through it to release the oats' benefits. Put fresh or dried lavender, rosemary, mint, marigold and/or chamomile in the bag for a divinely scented bath.

For baby-soft skin when you come out of the tub, try adding 500–750ml/17–25fl oz/2–3 cups of fresh milk to your bathwater. Milk and its derivatives contain lactic acid, which is a natural exfoliant. You will have to clean the tub very well after the bath, but your softer skin will make it worth the trouble, and although your skin will feel slightly oily, it will also be more supple. Use skimmed milk in your bath if you prefer less oily after-effects.

Sensual scented bath

Traditional Eastern spas are resplendent in the heady white blossoms that grow in abundance in the heat. The flowers' opulent scents evoke memories and emotions, and warm up the senses in every way. Used for thousands of years in closely guarded beauty recipes from India and Egypt to Indonesia and Thailand, the warm, rich aromas of jasmine, ylang-ylang and neroli are sensual and enticing, and blend beautifully together and with other essential oils.

Night-blooming jasmine, or Queen of the Night, has a wonderful fragrance that stimulates the senses. This expensive and rare oil has been used as an aphrodisiac for hundreds of years. Ylang-ylang has a heady floral aroma; by itself, it is sweet, but combined with other warm essential oils it creates beautifully exotic blends. Neroli, or orange blossom, is a tiny white flower that historically has symbolized purity. Its distinctive aroma instils calm.

For an exquisite tropical floral bath, place five drops each of ylang-ylang and sandalwood, three drops of jasmine and two drops of neroli essential oils in a glass jar and add two tablespoons of base oil, such as jojoba or almond. Shake the jar well to combine all the ingredients, and add to your bathwater, or massage into your body while your skin is still damp from bathing. Any remaining mixture can be stored in the jar.

Deep sea soak

The oceans, and the plants that grow within them, are so rich in minerals that any seaweed- or seawater-based body treatments are fabulous for making dry skin feel rejuvenated. The theory is that the chemical composition of seawater is almost identical to human plasma and therefore contains all the elements necessary for boosting cell renewal. Likewise, seaweed has a rich abundance of all the building blocks of life: minerals (such as sodium and potassium, which regulate fluid levels), trace elements (such as iodine, which regulates the metabolism, and iron, which improves circulation), amino acids, vitamins and a host of other nutrients.

So, turn the temperature up, turn the lights down low and keep a cup of iced water or fennel tea to hand to sip throughout the 20 minutes that you soak. This will encourage your body to flush out toxins and help reduce water retention and improve cellulite.

Ensure you choose a marine-based algae or seaweed solution from a reputable company for your bath. Lie with your body submerged for a full 20 minutes, to allow the marine water to draw out impurities and your body to absorb vitamins and minerals from the solution. Apply moisturizer to your skin when you emerge from the water in order to seal all the moisture within.

If you have a showerhead, try a light hydrotherapy treatment after your sea soak. This gently mimics ferocious jet spa treatments that further boost your circulation. Empty your tub and then stand up and vigorously spray your body with 10-second bursts of alternating cold and very warm water, focusing on your hip and thigh area. Repeat 10 times. Finish with a spray of warm water.

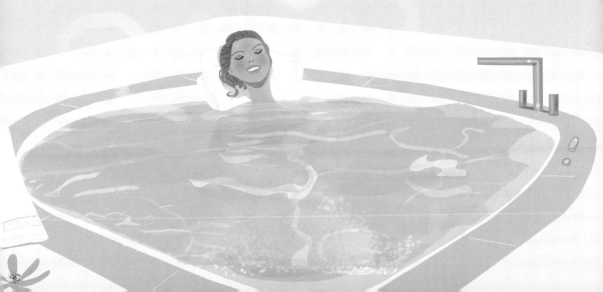

Seaweed shower treatment

Seaweed has a remarkable softening, remineralizing, moisturizing and firming effect on the skin. Applications of seaweeds help to detoxify the tissues and regulate blood circulation throughout the body. Seaweed supplies three essential skin health needs: it quenches free radicals with its beta-carotene, it improves skin colour and tone, and it reduces the effects of ageing. So, if you are interested in turning back the clock on your skin, a seaweed body treatment is a most pleasurable way to do so.

◆ Mix up a seaweed mask using 115g/4oz clay, 115g/4oz powdered kelp, 50g/2oz Spirulina powder and 20 drops of your favourite essential oil and store in an airtight container. Mix 75g/3oz of this mixture with enough hot water to make a paste, then brush or rub this over your entire body. Wrap yourself in a warm sheet for 15–20 minutes.

Wash off the seaweed mask in a bath, and rev up your circulation at the same time by using your showerhead as a spa-like jet spray and alternating the temperature from quite hot to cold.

To complete your treatment, throw 1kg/2lb 4oz of Dead Sea salts into your bathwater for a reviving yet relaxing soak.

Mud wrap

The healing properties of oceanic mud and clay have been used for centuries to cleanse and detoxify the body, and are rich in minerals that are easily absorbed by the skin. Great for times when your body feels jaded and stressed, a spa mud body wrap involves being slathered in warm mud or clay and then wrapped in layers of foil or plastic wrap, to help draw out toxins from the body. A few words of warning though: this treatment can get messy, and is best tried out in an empty bath.

Therapeutic clay or mud can be bought at any good health-food shop. For this treatment you will also need a couple of old towels, an old sheet, old blankets and ideally a climber's insulating reflective "space" blanket, if you can get one. The more body heat you can trap, the more beneficial it will be for your skin.

Spread out layers of a space blanket, blankets, towels and an old sheet. Mix the mud or clay paste according to the instructions (usually by adding water). Remove your bathrobe, apply the paste to your bottom and as much of your back as you can reach, then lie on the sheet and apply the paste to the rest of your body. Wrap yourself in the sheet first, followed by the towels, then the blankets and finally the space blanket. Tuck your arms in last of all, then lie back and relax for 20 minutes while the mud dries.

Then, unwrap yourself and remove the layers from the bath, carefully bunching them up so that no mud drops on to the floor. Rinse the mud off with warm water. Pat your skin dry and apply a rich body moisturizer.

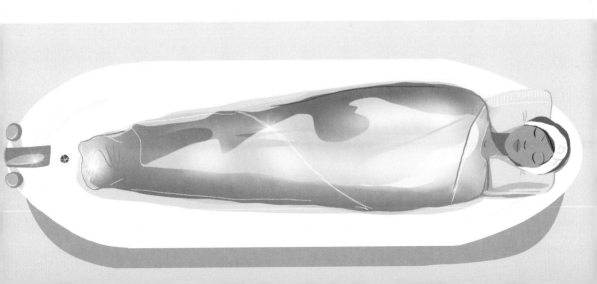

Body oil wrap

A body oil wrap is strictly a once-a-week all-over body treat. It takes a little while to arrange, so allow yourself the time, and don't be rushed. This treatment offers 30 minutes pure R&R and is a great way to wind down from the stresses of the day.

To start with, why not whip up your own blissed-out oil blend? Take two table-spoons of any combination of base oils such as olive, jojoba or almond, then add five drops each of anti-stress frankincense and vetiver essential oils (feel free to choose a different combination of calming oils if you prefer). Store your blend in a dark glass bottle to keep the aroma fresh to use at any time.

★ Warm a generous amount of oil between the palms of your hands. Beginning with the soles of your feet, massage it all over your body.

Put on an old bathrobe that you don't mind getting oily and stained, and put on old socks that you've warmed on a radiator. Now wrap yourself up cosily in several layers of blankets or a duvet, and lie down comfortably in a dimly lit room, perhaps with a few scented candles to create more atmosphere. Leave your body oil wrap on for at least 30 minutes, or overnight if possible.

Rose heaven

No flower is more instantly recognizable and no aroma more evocative than that of the rose. Its rich fragrance has perfumed our history for generations, from ancient Persian gardens to extravagant Roman banquets, and the flower has long symbolized innocence, love, passion and luxury all at once. Rose oil is mood-enhancing, yet calming to the skin and the senses, making it the perfect oil to choose in times of stress. Its aroma is powerful but comforting, and likewise rose is toning and balancing for the skin. Rose oil suits all skin types, but especially sensitive, dry and mature skin.

◆ Spritz a little rosewater over your face, shoulders and body. Add 10 drops of rose absolute essential oil to two tablespoons of almond oil, then add six drops of this blend to a cupful of unscented body lotion.

Diffuse two drops of the same blend with one drop of frankincense essential oil in an oil burner or a vaporizer. Sit very comfortably; then, starting with your hands and your feet, smooth the oil blend over your body, working inward toward the heart with small circular strokes.

Wrap yourself up warmly in a big fluffy bathrobe and bed socks, or even lie under a duvet, for 15–20 minutes while the oil is absorbed, then apply the rose-scented body lotion in exactly the same way. Wrap up again, then climb back under the duvet and relax for another 15–20 minutes.

Fake tan

One foolproof way to look as if you've been lounging around a tropical beach spa is to fake a tan. There's no denying that glowing, honey-gold skin makes us look much lighter and healthier than pale, greyish skin. But, as we all know, it's much safer to get it from a bottle than to get it from the sun. Today's self-tanning products provide an authentic-looking tan without any of the sun's harmful effects.

If you've never used a self-tanning product before, try this fool-proof application, which will ensure an even, healthy-looking tan on even the whitest of skins. If you're still not convinced, buy a self-tan product designed for the face and use it on your body (lighter still) or one of the new style progressive fake tans that build up day by day. Do practise applying them a few times, especially if you are very pale, and never try out a new formula the day before an important occasion or going on holiday.

◆ Start by exfoliating your whole body. Pay particular attention to areas of dry skin such as the knees and elbows, which otherwise tend to absorb more tanning cream and end up looking darker. Then apply body lotion to these areas, to act as a slight barrier. Allow 5–10 minutes for it to be absorbed.

Next, apply self-tan all over your body, massaging it in evenly. Wash your hands immediately. Being careful not to touch anything, let the self-tan dry on your skin for at least 15 minutes (or as instructed by the brand you chose).

Allow one hour, then, regardless of how long the brand says to wait, take a shower. This ensures that any colour that hasn't been absorbed by this point will wash away, so you are less likely to end up with streaky uneven patches.

Spa pedicure

This mini spa pedicure will transform your feet, leaving them moisturized, soothed and blissfully relaxed. Choose a comfortable chair and make sure you have all the items and ingredients you need to hand. In a bowl mix five tablespoons of jojoba, almond or olive oil, five drops of lemon essential oil or lemon juice and two table-spoons of sugar. Fill a footbath or large bowl with warm water, add four tablespoons of base oil and place the bowl on a towel on the floor. Wet two small towels and warm them in a microwave, then place them in a plastic bag for later use.

◆ Remove any old nail polish. Trim your nails and file them into your desired shape. Place your feet in the footbath for 10 minutes and relax. Bliss! Now dry your feet and push your cuticles back with an orange stick.

Next, apply the lemon and sugar scrub to your feet, making sure every area is treated. Rinse off with the water from the footbath, then dry your feet and gently massage some oil or cream (cuticle cream if you have it) into the nails and cuticles. Wrap the warm towels around your feet and leave on until the heat fades. Rub a foot file on any rough areas, such as your heels.

Finally, massage in a little lotion or oil (preferably almond oil) to seal in the moisture before painting your nails.

Hair pack

Parched, dry, dehydrated hair is extremely porous and soon becomes dull and life-less. A nourishing treatment can replace moisture and suppleness, making your hair shinier and easier to manage and style. Hair masks are time-consuming, but set aside an hour to do the treatment properly, and you won't believe the difference in your hair, especially if it is mid-length to long, which is the driest.

Olive oil makes a simple but effective hair mask. It nourishes, conditions and improves the strength and elasticity of your hair, improving its manageablility and health. A hair mask will also cleanse and invigorate your scalp, helping to create better looking hair and improve any stressful scalp conditions.

This conditioning hair pack will add lustre. Mix one egg to one part mayonnaise and one part olive oil, and apply to your hair. Cover your hair in clear plastic wrap and then in a towel, and allow the pack to work for at least 30 minutes. Rinse out, then shampoo and condition as usual. You'll find your hair is smooth, with renewed shine.

For an aromatic treatment, combine 125ml/4fl oz/½ cup olive oil and five drops of frankincense essential oil in a lidded jar. Shake well and leave for 24 hours in a cool dark place. Rinse your hair with warm water. Shake the mixture, then warm one tablespoon of it in the palms of your hands. Massage into your scalp using your fingertips to make tiny circles (see page 47). Repeat until you've massaged your entire scalp. Rub the ends of your hair with any remaining oil (if there's a lot left over, keep it for the next application). Place a plastic bag over your hair and scalp and leave for at least half an hour. Rinse well, then shampoo as usual.

Relaxing facial

Facials are one of the most popular of all spa treatments, but you can easily give yourself a blissfully relaxing facial at home in half an hour, with just a few aromatic ingredients. Facials can help to improve and maintain your skin tone for longer as well as helping to keep your skin clear of impurities.

This is a relaxing activity, so make sure you have everything you need to hand (including all your facial products and a muslin facecloth), and allow plenty of time. Choose the right venue for your facial: a bedroom with nearby bathroom is ideal, as you will need water and a place to lie down while the facemask is on. Pat your skin dry between each step with fresh tissues and use this time to look more closely at your skin, getting to know it a little bit better.

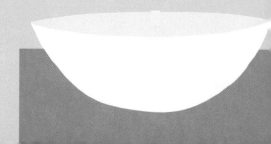

◆ Warm some cleanser between the palms of your hands, then massage it into your skin with firm, circular movements. If it's a creamy cleanser, blot any excess with a tissue, then wipe off the remaining cream. If you use a rinse-off cleanser, splash your face with clean water, and finally remove any residue with a damp muslin facecloth or flannel.

Next, fill a bowl with hot water, then add a few fresh herbs such as lavender, basil or rosemary, or add one drop of each of the essential oils of these herbs. Lean over the bowl with your face in the steam and drape a towel over both your head and the bowl. Stay like this, breathing deeply, for up to five minutes, depending on how sensitive your skin is and how comfortable you are.

The next part of your relaxing facial is an exfoliation, followed by the application of a toner and then a facemask. You conclude your treatment with a gentle massage using a facial oil. This massage will brighten your complexion, and help to detoxify your skin by activating pressure points to improve the lymphatic drainage around your face. Use a calming blend of two drops each of rose and lavender oils in two teaspoons of almond oil.

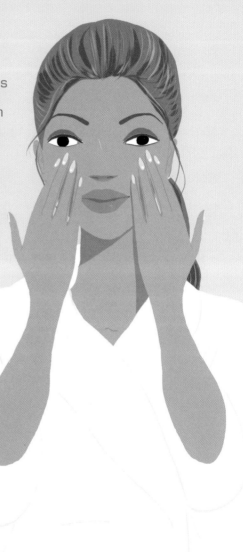

◆ Gently exfoliate your skin with a scrub or a muslin facecloth, to buff away any dead skin cells that have been loosened. Rinse thoroughly with warm water. Next, tone your skin with rosewater, either in a spray as a spritzer or smoothed over your skin on cotton wool pads.

Next, apply a facemask (see pages 58–61) suitable for how your skin looks and feels. Close your eyes and lie back for 10 minutes, or however long instructed. Remove, using your muslin facecloth to get the last traces off your skin.

Start your face massage by placing your fingers on both eyebrows. Press slowly, then release. Repeat this three times. Then move the position of your fingers to just under your eyes and again, with light and slow pressure, press and release three times. Then sweep your fingertips up to the centre of your forehead and press outward toward your temples on either side. Pressing along your hairline, move past your cheekbones, pinching your earlobes, and press along your jaw line until your fingertips finally meet at your chin.

To finish your facial, blot off excess oil with a clean tissue, then apply your usual moisturizer or night cream.

Spa brow makeover

Eyebrows are an underrated part of your face. The arch, shape and width of your brows all influence your facial expression, making you appear cross, curious, older or even younger. If you make up your eyes but neglect your brows, your face simply looks "unfinished". However, neat, defined brows are flattering to your eyes, opening them up and enhancing their shape. So, even if you do nothing else for the day, sit yourself down at a mirror in daylight, with a great new set of tweezers, and get ready to restyle your face.

◆ First define the limits of your brows. Hold a pencil along the side of your nose. Your brow's thicker inner edge should start vertically above the inner corner of your eye. Now swing the top of the pencil to the outer corner of your eye; your brow should end in a diagonal line with it. The arch of your brow should be just beyond the outer edge of your iris.

To shape your brows properly, always pluck one hair at a time from underneath the natural brow line. Never pluck hairs from above your brow line, or your brows may end up patchy and unbalanced. If the hairs from the inner edge of your brow (by your nose) to the brow arch are long, brush them straight up and trim them into line with the top of your brow.

If your brows are pale, thin or sparse, fill them in with a brow pencil or powder. The colour should match the natural shade of your brows or be a tone lighter, but never darker. Brush through using a stiff brow brush, working the colour upward and outward, following the shape of your natural brow line.

Inner cleanse

Does your skin look dull and lifeless? Do you wake up in the morning feeling tired and hung-over, even though you went to bed early? If so, it's time to take steps to cancel out all the detrimental effects of modern living and treat your body to a complete cleansing regime with a spa liver detox.

Three days before starting your detox, eliminate processed foods, caffeine, red meat and alcohol from your diet, and drink at least 2 litres/3½ pints/8 cups of mineral water per day. Plan on doing a liver detox over a weekend, because you may feel tired, or suffer from diarrhoea or stomach cramps. If you find this liver flush unpleasant, consult your pharmacist who can recommend suitable supplements instead. Ensure that you consult your doctor if you have any physical problems, and do not do a liver flush if you are pregnant or breastfeeding.

This two-day liver flush technique is used by a number of complementary medicine practitioners.

In a jug or bowl, mix four teaspoons of Epsom salts with ½ teaspoon of vitamin C powder in 750ml/1¼ pints/3 cups of water. This makes up four servings of "Epsom mix".

In a separate jar mix 125ml/4fl oz/½ cup of olive oil and 50ml/2 fl oz/¼ cup each of squeezed grapefruit juice and squeezed lemon juice. Shake briskly until well blended.

On the morning of day one, drink the first serving of the Epsom mix. Two hours later, drink a second serving; then, 1¾ hours later, shake the oil mixture and drink half of it. Repeat this process on day two.

Spa fast

Spas are increasingly renowned for their detox programmes: diets and cleansing systems devoted to clearing your body of the residue of your lifestyle and giving it a "spring clean". The main idea behind detoxification is to help the body eliminate substances that it may have accumulated over time that are "toxic" to our health. These can come from the environment, or from the food we ingest. Most of them are dealt with naturally by the body, but from time to time the systems that clear toxins may not work as efficiently as they should.

The best, and simplest, way to detox is to follow a raw fruit and vegetable diet for a few days. In addition to detoxifying your system and flushing out your colon, a diet like this will improve your energy levels, increase your ability to concentrate and may even enhance your enjoyment of and outlook on life.

◆ The raw diet, as its name implies, is based on consuming unprocessed, ideally organic, whole plant-based foods, at least 75 per cent of which should be uncooked. It mainly consists of fresh fruit and vegetables, nuts and seeds, beans, grains, legumes, dried fruits, seaweeds, sun-dried fruits, freshly made fruit and vegetable juices and purified water.

Followers of a raw diet cite numerous long-term health benefits, including increased energy levels, improved digestion, better skin, weight loss, and stronger immune systems.

Detox on a weekend or when your schedule is not too demanding, as you may experience fatigue, headaches, aching muscles, unsettled moods or emotions, diarrhoea and skin breakouts – all of which are encouraging signs that your body is detoxifying.

De-stress massage

Nothing beats massage when it comes to stimulating the whole body, helping to exhilarate the senses, ease emotions and soothe the soul. Favourite de-stressing massage techniques are: effleurage, a light stroke over the body in a rhythmic pattern; kneading, more of a gentle pinch to activate nerve endings; and palming, which creates warmth in the skin as you press the palm over the same area again and again. I suggest you "feel your way" – trust your own innate sense of what feels relaxing and enjoyable to create a massage technique you truly enjoy.

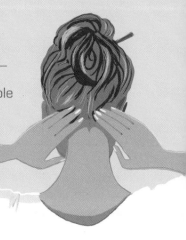

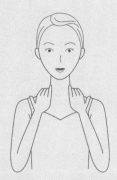 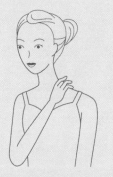 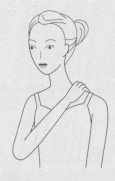

1 Warm a little almond oil between your hands and smooth it onto your neck and shoulders. Press and rotate the fingers of each hand into the muscles at the base of your neck on either side of the spine, and work up to the base of your skull. Move to the sides of your neck and repeat, alternating between firm and gentle pressure.

2 Next, work over your shoulders. Using your fingertips, tap and press firmly along your shoulder from your neck to the top of your arms. You can also press using the flat of your hands, or alternate between the two techniques, depending on which sensation you prefer. Work back and forth along your shoulders to the neck for several minutes.

3 Finish by squeezing your shoulder muscles between your fingers and the heel of your hand to relieve blockages of tension.

Inner spa bliss

It's great to lavish your body with extra attention and care, but it's also important to nurture your inner self. While up to now you've focused on the way you look to make you feel more positive about yourself, in this chapter you will explore a variety of ways to help you become a calmer, more peaceful, more delightful person, who is happier and therefore easier to be around. The best thing about experiencing a bit of spa bliss is that you'll emerge feeling as if you are far more in control and content with the person you are.

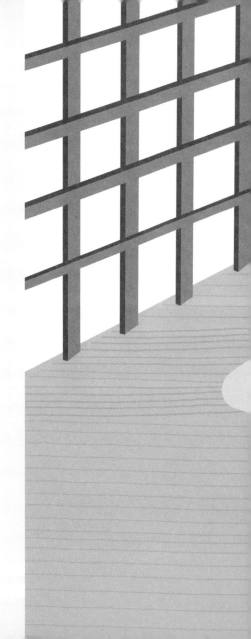

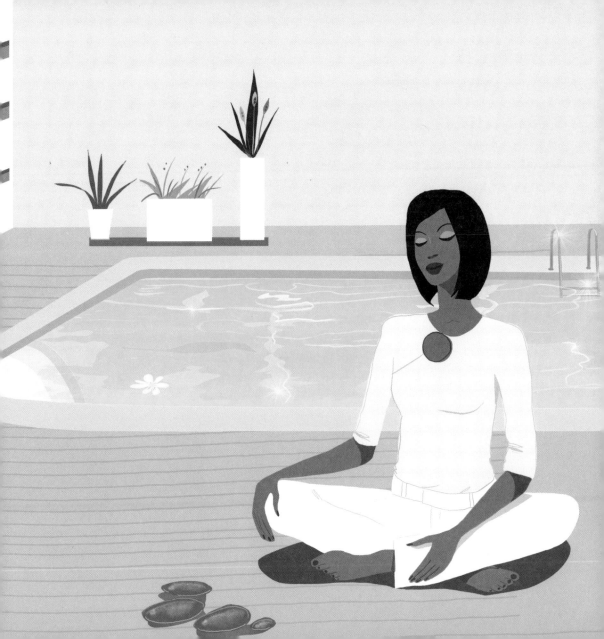

Love your body

Think more positively about who you are. You are what you believe yourself to be: just as you are what you eat, so you are what you think. Practise positive thoughts (called "affirmations") and associations and learn to appreciate the fullness of your life in every aspect. Try to develop a "diva attitude": smile as much as possible and, when you look at your reflection in the mirror, tell yourself, "I am beautiful." If you continually think negative things about yourself, this will undoubtedly be reflected in the image you project to others. Learn to talk to yourself in positive terms and you will end up having greater self-belief.

Research has found that women who think of themselves as beautiful are much more successful than those with a poor body image, partly as a result of their high self-esteem. But look at the wording carefully: you only need to think of yourself as beautiful, not necessarily be beautiful.

Look at yourself in a mirror. Gaze uninterrupted at your reflection for a few minutes in silence, and use this time to make positive affirmations. Repeating the same statements helps to reinforce the way you want to feel and can create renewed confidence and improved self-awareness, leading to more contentment. Try one of these affirmations, or make up your own:

To calm down: "I breathe slowly, I relax my muscles."

To be more confident: "I let go of worry when I make mistakes. I sense what is right for me. I dwell on positive things. I am worthy and I value myself."

For self-belief: "I trust in my abilities. I nurture myself. I have self-respect. Others sense my positive energy."

Visualization ritual

Visualization is the art of relaxation through mental imagery. Both positive and negative pictures are constantly flooding through our brains, and these can have a profound effect on our entire being, physically, mentally, emotionally and spiritually. Through visualization, we can lean how to harness the power of these images for good. Phobia sufferers can imagine themselves confronting their fears; cancer patients can picture their healthy cells overcoming the malignant cells; and shy people can see themselves as happy and confident. Focusing on positive images can help to bring the reality into being. Once you get the hang of it, visualization enhances any deep-breathing ritual and can boost all your spa treatments.

◆ Make yourself comfortable. This may be lying propped up on cushions in a candlelit room, sitting in your favourite armchair or lying back in a warm bath. Once you are breathing deeply and regularly, close your eyes and focus your mind on somewhere you find beautiful, happy or peaceful. This can be anywhere that is particular to you and gives you positive feelings: on a pristine, remote beach, in a tranquil blue sea, in a warm tropical rainforest, or in a colourful, fresh spring garden.

Make a mental picture of everything the way it was when you were there: the warmth of the sun on your skin, the light, the scenery, the peace and happiness you felt … and then imagine yourself there again. Keep your breathing deep and regular and stay like this for at least 20 minutes, or however long you are comfortable.

Restful breathing ritual

It's our first instinct when we are born, and it's fundamental to every living cell in our body, so you'd think by now we'd know how to breathe properly. Yet so many of us use less than half our total lung capacity when we breathe. Worse still, when we're stressed we resort to shallow breathing, which only makes us more anxious. You have probably found that the people you have met who practise yoga, T'ai Chi or Pilates are generally more focused and calm in their approach to life – and this may be partly due to their breath control. So why not learn how to breathe deeply and rhythmically? It need only take 5–10 minutes a day, but it can have a profound effect on your mood and your approach to daily life.

Lie on your back (on a mat if you wish), arms and legs stretched out slightly, palms facing upward and toes facing out. Concentrate on relaxing all your limbs, feeling your spine settle.

Place your hands lightly on your lower abdomen. Take a deep breath in through your nose. Keep your body relaxed as your lungs fill with air and your lower abdomen rises. Then breathe out through your mouth as your tummy falls. Focus only on the rise and fall of your hands in tune with your breathing. Breathe in and out like this 10 times.

Next, place your hands at the base of your ribs. Breathe in, keeping your shoulders and arms relaxed, and feel your breath through your fingertips as your ribs stretch and open. Breathe deeply and slowly for 10 breaths.

Finally, place your hands on your sternum. Hold here, and again breathe in deeply and feel in rhythm and at peace with your precious breath.

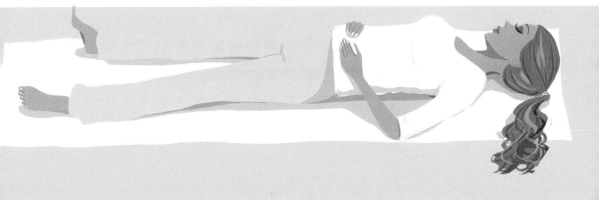

Meditation ritual

Meditation is the ultimate mind, body and soul therapy. Research consistently shows that meditation can slow the heart rate and breathing, lower blood pressure, boost the immune system and reduce muscle tension and headaches, all of which are linked to stress-related illnesses. Meditation also clears the mind, giving you new focus and vigour, and power – mind power – from within.

First you need to empty your mind of its constant daily chatter. One way of doing this is to concentrate on one single thing, which can be whatever works for you. Try meditating on a crystal, such as rose quartz, which is used in crystal healing to create a loving and peaceful atmosphere. Sit comfortably with a rose quartz crystal in your hands. Close your eyes and focus on the colour of the crystal in your mind. Imagine love and peace radiating from your heart and the crystal into the world around you. Breathe deeply and stay here for as long as you like.

◆ Sit comfortably, close your eyes and breathe slowly and deeply for a few minutes. Now imagine a white light entering your body through the very top of your head. As it does so, allow your head to become filled with light, then visualize letting the light flood down your spine and filter out into your arms and legs, fingertips and toes.

Now focus your mind on this light travelling back the way it came, pausing occasionally as it travels toward your head. Allow the light to form a colour where it rests. Once the light reaches the top of your head, gently let it out. When you have finished, sit for a moment, then gradually open your eyes. Stay still for a moment longer, then move on with your day.

Morning yoga

Yoga is the ancient practice that combines relaxation and exercise for mind, body and spirit. This adapted version of a classic sun salutation, that will take you just five minutes to practise, stretches every muscle group in your body. This will stimulate your energy flow, so it is the perfect exercise for first thing in the morning. Practise the sequence of exercises illustrated opposite and on page 111 until the movements flow together seamlessly.

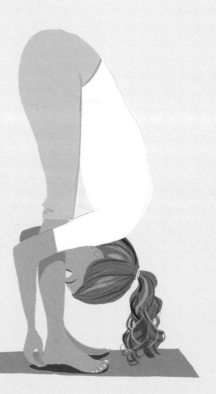

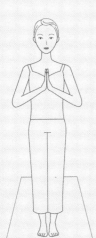

1 Stand upright with your shoulders relaxed, your back straight, tummy in, feet together and hands at chest level in prayer position. Take four or five deep breaths through your nose.

2 Breathe in through your nose and breathe out again as you stretch your arms above your head.

3 Breathe out as you bend forward from your hips, reaching down to the floor with your fingertips. Hold your ankles, bringing your head as close to your legs as feels comfortable.

The postures (or asanas) that make up this sun salutation are gentle stretches that will improve your balance, strength and flexibility, complemented with breathing techniques. The movements are slow and controlled – try to think of yourself as entering, holding and releasing each pose. They work on the entire body, including the internal organs, which are massaged by specific movements.

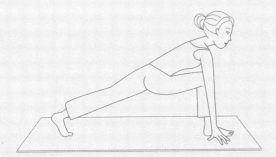

4 Place your hands on the floor in front of you, breathe in and stretch your left leg back, toes tucked under, as you bend your right knee to a right-angle. (If you aren't yet flexible enough, keep your left leg slightly bent at the knee so that you don't over-stretch yourself.)

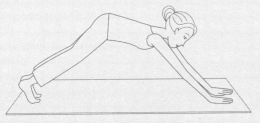

5 Breathe out as you extend your right leg back too, feet hip-width apart, then push down through your hands, swing your hips upward and back and move your chest toward your knees. Bring your head down between your arms.

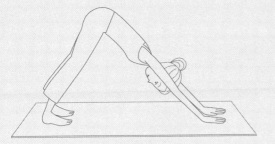

6 Push your hips further into the air to create an upside-down "V" shape with your body. Breathe in, step your feet between your hands and bring your arms over your head as you come back up to standing tall, then bring your hands back to prayer position.

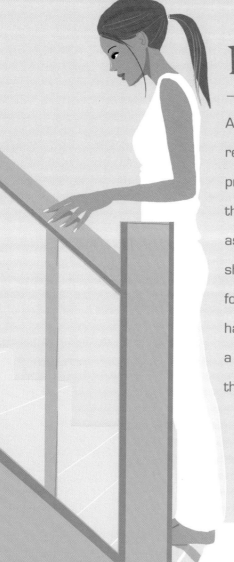

Restful routine

Apart from keeping you flexible, strong and lean, regular exercise such as this mini spa workout provides a long-lasting feel-good factor through the release in your brain of natural opiates known as endorphins. To keep yourself fit and well, you should aim to exercise at least three times a week for a minimum of 20 minutes at a time. Research has shown that consistent moderate exercise over a longer period of time burns fat more effectively than shorter, more intense workouts.

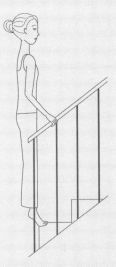

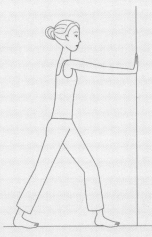

1 To work your lower legs, stand in front of a low step, such as the lowest stair on a staircase. Put the balls of your feet on the step and press into them to rise up. Then release to lower down again. Repeat 12 times.

Tucking in your tummy strengthens your abdominal muscles, which in turn stabilizes your back and improves your posture, making you look taller and slimmer. When you have a few minutes, pull in your tummy, hold it for a count of three, then let it go. Repeat 12 times.

2 To stretch and engage your leg muscles and tone your arms, stand in front of a wall, with your feet hip-width apart. Place your palms on the wall and step your right leg about 30cm/1ft behind you. Bend your left knee and feel the stretch in your right leg; as you do so, bend your arms. Straighten your knee and your arms at the same time. Repeat the exercise three times, then swap legs so that your right foot is in front, and repeat three times.

Clear the air

Positively charged ions in the air may be one of the reasons why we often feel tired and lethargic (especially when we're trying to get up in the morning). Although positive ions sound good, they are believed to contribute to a number of common ailments including migraines, headaches and breathing difficulties. To tackle them, we need to surround ourselves and our homes with more negatively charged ions, which are invigorating rather than energy-sapping.

I recommend buying an ionizer and placing it near your bed. It will pump out healthy negative ions into your bedroom environment, helping you to breathe and sleep more easily. If you keep the central heating on at night, balance a saucer of water (perhaps with a few drops of rebalancing lavender essential oil in it) on top of the bedroom radiator, or invest in a humidifier to add some moisture to the air.

◆ Air is all around us. It's the element of spring, of newness, awakening and enlightenment. If we want to change the way we feel, or are seeking focus, romance or inspiration, then vaporizing essential oils into the room to create a positive ambience is a great thing to do. It's especially beneficial if you are planning to practise some deep breathing or meditation techniques.

Simply use an aromatherapy burner to warm your chosen essential oil, or an electrical diffuser to blow air around the oil. You can also make your own aroma-therapy spray: add six drops of essential oils to fresh water in a plant misting bottle, and use like an air freshener. Try combining rose and geranium oils for a soft, sensual, feminine aroma to envelop yourself in. Bliss!

Flower essences to calm

In the 1930s, Dr Edward Bach discovered that if plants were floated in water in full sunlight or moonlight, the flowers would energize the water with their molecular imprint. The healing properties of these "flower essences" are now acknowledged around the world. The principle of flower essences is that they resonate with our own energy and thereby balance our emotions, treating issues such as grief, anger or low self-esteem, that can eventually result in physical complaints if ignored. Flower essence makers produce fresh batches of essences that, when you take them orally as prescribed by a therapist, you may feel as a shift in energy. Here are my favourite flower remedies for bliss.

◆ Stargazer lily allows energy to flow freely, soothing any emotions that may be holding back your creativity and increasing positive feelings of love and self-worth.

Self heal relaxes the mind and triggers awareness of where true healing may lie or be required. It is powerfully restorative, but can cause you to reveal or admit more than you would like.

St John's wort works with your "fight-or-flight" response, helping you to stand your ground or to escape effectively, depending on what is appropriate. It is a fabulous essence for quiet, shy people who would like to be more assertive.

Magnolia improves clear-thinking and intuition and will help you develop a more proactive attitude.

Motherwort also works on the intuition, helping to eliminate negativity. It brings a better balance to personal relationships.

Agrimony inspires spiritual awareness and wisdom. It will give you the courage to face difficult situations.

Rest easy

Just be. Sometimes when you feel overloaded by life, the best thing is to take a step back from your daily routine. A positive outlook frees the mind, body and spirit, but it may be that only by letting go can you see the big picture.

You've been pampered and cosseted, now just relax and let the joy of living come into your life each day, and you will feel both renewed and energized. Seek and find your true sense of worth, to rekindle your spirit and enliven your soul.

◆ Learn ways of overcoming both the causes and the effects of stress on your mind and body. Armed with this ability for self-control, you will achieve so much more.

Seek less perfection in yourself. If you focus on your positive aspects, you will reduce how often you automatically criticize yourself. Your positive attitude will then be reflected in the way others perceive and relate to you.

Write down how you feel, both about the areas in your life you're happy with and those that may be causing tension and stress. Writing down your thoughts helps to create clarity and can make you all the more realistic about problems and determined about solutions.

Most of all, enjoy and take pleasure from this book. *Spa Bliss* is all about getting the best from yourself, discovering a new you from the inside out.

Spa sessions

Here is a selection of spa pampering sequences, made up of different combinations of treatments in this book that work well together. I've designed each sequence to suit a specific purpose, such as all-over relaxation or tackling problematic hair, and I have also put together a spa session that you can try out over a weekend.

These sequences and sessions are an ideal way to organize your escape from the hustle and bustle of everyday life. Of course, you can adapt these suggested sessions as you choose; feel free to add and subtract treatments depending on your situation and how much time you have. For any of these sequences, it's helpful to plan ahead and make sure you have all the ingredients you may need. Finally, don't forget to put yourself into the zone – make sure you're not going to be disturbed, turn off the phone and take time out from your world to enjoy your spa bliss!

De-stress Express

- De-stress massage
- Eye restore
- Fruit soother
- Hand massage

All Over Body Bliss

- Salt glow scrub
- Deep sea soak
- Body oil wrap
- Foot massage

Use this sequence when you need to find relaxation fast. Start by smoothing away tension from your face as shown on page 29. Soothe your eyes with tea bags (page 31), and calm your insides too with a juice (page 33). Finally, a gentle hand massage is a sure-fire stress reliever (page 51).

This sequence will restore your body to glowing, gorgeous health. Slough away dead skin cells with an exfoliating scrub (page 43), and then revive your skin with a magical mineral-laden bath (page 71). Relax with a sensual body oil wrap (page 77) and an uplifting foot massage (page 55).

Scalp and Brow Refresher

- Hair and scalp massage
- Hair pack
- Frown anti-age massage
- Spa brow makeover

This sequence will leave your hair and scalp beautifully refreshed, and your brows neat and tidy. First stimulate your hair and scalp with a massage (page 47), before applying a hair pack (page 85). While the hair pack works, tidy your brows (page 91), and finish with an anti-age massage (page 45).

Weekend Spa Session

Clear your social schedule and turn your home into a spa for the weekend. Why not invite some girlfriends over to share the spa experience with you? Make sure you have plenty of healthy food and drink in the house to prevent stressful trips to the supermarket.

Take a little extra time over these two days to focus on your internal as well as your external well-being. Include meditation and exercise activities along with your beauty treatments, and make sure you deeply relax.

Day 1

- Relaxing facial
- Restful tummy massage
- Blissful spa bath
- Meditation ritual

A full facial (pages 87 and 89) will enliven your skin and get the weekend off to a great start. A soothing tummy massage (page 49) should get you in the mood for a therapeutic spa bath (page 65). Close your day of pampering with a meditative ritual (page 107), ensuring a good night's sleep.

Day 2

- Morning yoga
- Rose heaven
- Spa manicure
- Spa pedicure

Start Day 2 with a yoga routine (pages 109 and 111) to revive your muscles, then treat your senses with a delicious rose body treatment (page 79). Groom hands and feet with a spa manicure (page 53) and pedicure (page 83), and you'll return to the world looking and feeling completely refreshed.

Useful resources

If you'd like to experience exotic spa treatments and rituals a little further, there's a wealth of resources available from books and CDs to put you in the mood even more. Here are a few of my personal favourites.

BOOKS

Christopher Hansard, *The Tibetan Art of Positive Thinking: Skilful Thoughts for Successful Living* (Hodder & Stoughton, 2003)

Christopher Hansard, *The Tibetan Art of Living: Wise Body, Wise Mind, Wise Life* (Hodder Mobius, 2002)

Louise L. Hay, *You Can Heal Your Life* (Hay House, US 1998)

Kathy Phillips, *The Spirit of Yoga* (Hachette Illustrated, UK 2005)

Barbara Olive, *The Flower Healer* (Cico Books, UK 2007)

Lesley Garner, *Everything I've Ever Done That Worked*
(Hay House, UK 2004)

Dr Leslie Baumann, *The Skin Type Solution*
(Hodder & Stoughton, 2006)

CDs

David Naegele, *Temple in the Forest*
(Valley of the Sun, 1985)

Dean Evenson, *Forest Rain*
(Soundings of the Planet, 1993)

Ben Leinbach, *The Spirit of Yoga*
(Real Music, 2002)

Gurudass, *Flowers in the Rain*
(Spirit Voyage Music, 2007)

Index